LUPUS DIET

Written by

Nick Bishopton

TABLE OF CONTENTS

INTRODUCTION

What is Lupus and how can an appropriate diet help?

Lupus is a chronic inflammatory disease that affects the immune system causing the immune system to attack healthy cells, tissue and organs in the body and subsequently setting off a cascade of events leading to widespread inflammation in the whole body. It can be triggered by a number of factors which are yet to be fully explained, but in simple terms the immune system mistakenly attacks the body's own healthy tissue.

However, research has been able to identify that genetics and an individual's diet and lifestyle play different roles in triggering the inflammatory process. When lupus occurs in the body, there exists a high level of persistent inflammation which affects those very delicate organs of the body such as the endocrine glands, brain, heart, kidneys, lungs and joints.

Often lupus is also called SLE, which is an abbreviation for Systemic Lupus Erythematosus. Statistics have shown that women are affected ten times more than men due to the presence of up surging hormones, 90% of cases are reported in women around the age of 30, but this disease can also occur in men and in children.

It is often difficult to diagnose SLE because its symptoms and that of other health conditions, such as Lyme disease, thyroid disorders and fibromyalgia, are similar. The following are potential causes of lupus: allergic reactions, emotional stress, viral diseases/infections, estrogen disruption etc. These can cause an immediate outburst of lupus.

Lupus is an auto immune condition and the symptoms can be worsened when the wrong foods or certain medications are ingested. There are many plans to help fight the disease and they involve the use of various medications, diet, life style modification, therapy, etc.

While lupus is treatable with medication, there is no way to prevent the disease. Also, these medications when taken can cause certain side effects. Thus in order to achieve optimum treatment, good nutrition is really important. Given that this disease is systemic, it is required that good nutritional habits are maintained helping the body to remain as healthy as possible.

Living with lupus requires you to consume certain foods to improve your life, whilst at the same time avoiding certain foods that can exacerbate the situation through increasing or triggering flares. Aim for a well balanced diet that contains anti oxidants such as plenty of fruits, vegetables and whole grains. To minimize the effects of inflammation on the body eat balanced meals, diets that are healthy for the heart, nutrient dense foods (lots of drugs make certain nutrients deficient in the body).

Anti oxidants mop up the oxidative contents formed in the blood by the inflammation. If you have lupus, the use of a varied, healthy diet will help in the reduction of inflammation and its symptoms, be effective in combating the unwanted effects of drugs used in treatment, have and maintain a healthy weight, ensure the maintenance of strong bones and muscles, reduce to a minimum the risks of having heart disease, increase your level of energy and maintain a healthy body weight and improve your bowel health.

LUPUS IN FOCUS

What is the disease?

As stated earlier, lupus is an autoimmune disease that causes the immune system to become hyperactive and subsequently attacking normal, healthy tissue. Also known as SLE (Systemic Lupus Erythematosus), this disease causes inflammation (swelling) which is the primary symptom along with many other symptoms. It is a chronic disease which implies that it doesn't go away, so it is a condition that you have to manage for the rest of your life.

The cause of SLE is yet to be understood though it is believed that genetics and various environmental factors such as exposure to ultraviolet rays, continuous use of certain medications play roles in starting off lupus in a human body. Research has postulated the feasibility of lupus being aggravated or precipitated by the aforementioned environmental factors as the immune system can be easily stimulated by them even with brief exposure.

Certain factors are also believed to be involved in the occurrence of the disease. Such factors include presence of female hormones, smoking, excess exposure to sunlight, deficiency of Vitamin D and viral infections.

Due to the presence of the reproductive hormones, women with SLE can also experience a worsening of their symptoms prior to menstruation. This backs up the fact that female hormones play a very important role in the higher likelihood of the occurrence of SLE in women than in men.

The failure of a certain key enzyme in disposing of dying cells explains the relationship between DNA/ genetics and lupus. Research showed that mutation of this gene required for the disposal of the dying cells contributes in the initiation of lupus.

There are certain medications that have been reported as a facilitator in the triggering of SLE. The drug induced lupus disease state comes about from the side effects of these drugs. The drugs include: hydralazine, phenytoin, quinidine, d-penicillamase and isoniazid.

While functioning properly, the body's immune system produces proteins referred to as antibodies which help to fight and protect against antigens such as viruses and bacteria. To avoid the occurrence of the flares that come with this disease, it is advised that people with the disease avoid sun exposures, monitor their condition with their doctor and avoid discontinuing their medications abruptly.

Because the accompanying inflaming cells and antibodies are able to affect any body tissues, this disease has the ability to affect any part of your body leading to the occurrence of diseases in such areas such as the heart, the skin, kidney, nervous system and even the joints. When it affects the skin and rashes break out, the state of the body at that moment is referred to as lupus dermatitis. This type of lupus occurs only on the skin without being systemic and this is referred to as being a discoid form of lupus. When the lupus penetrates into the internal organs on further neglect, the patient's state becomes a systemic form of the lupus disease.

These two forms of diseases occur 8 times less in men than in women, it affects all ages but mostly individuals of age between 21-46. In addition, this disease affects African Americans, citizens of Japanese and Chinese descent where their women are 4 times more likely to develop the disease that white women would. When it affects women from these countries at a younger age, several other problems arise such as kidney disease appearing.

Take note that lupus is said to be similar to cancer, as it has no causative microorganism that is infectious nor is it contagious. As such genetic factors play a high role in increasing the chances of autoimmune diseases developing in an individual. One can have lupus disease in his/her lineage and in addition have a high probability to suffer other auto immune diseases like autoimmune related thyroid disorders, and rheumatoid arthritis.

How does this effect people?

Given that female hormones play an important role in this disease, it can be easily summarized that this disease is a woman's health issue. That's not however the truth. And although women have a high prevalence of the disease it certainly effects many men.

Statistics show that about 10% of individuals who manifest lupus first on their skin will end up with systemic form of the disease. It often manifests as a characteristic facial flat, red painless rash which does not itch starting at the nose's bridge and can be referred to as the butterfly rash at this stage. The rash tends to worsen on exposure to the sun making such an individual photosensitive and this can be accompanied by an increase in inflammation all over the body.

At this stage, it is referred to having a "flare". The patient can start to experience other autoimmune diseases such as arthritis which can be misunderstood as rheumatoid arthritis. Also alopecia can set in with a consequent increase in the deteriorating rate of the patient's health.

What are the symptoms?

Derived from the latin word lupus, which means wolf, the first symptom often observed is the occurrence rash on the bridge of the nose which gradually spreads to the other parts of the face making the patient take on the face of a wolf. On the occurrence of the systemic form of the disease, other organ and tissue damages can occur. Other symptoms that can occur include: alopecia, low grade fever, arthritis, pericarditis, photosensitivity, muscle aches, nose and mouth ulcer, butterfly rash, pleuritis and Raynaud's phenomenon.

Depending on the level of organ involvement and disease severity, complications in these organs can further increase the symptoms. SLE associated manifestations on the skin can lead to the scarring of the skin. Given that skin rash can appear on both the scalp and face in a patient with discoid lupus, if not properly treated, scarring can occur on the head/scalp causing alopecia.

SLE depletes the percentage and content of white blood cells in the body. This in turn can cause thrombocytopenia, leading to the occurrence of spontaneous blood clotting, thrombosis and anemia (low blood cell count). The decrease in Leucocytes content can increase the occurrence of any infection while thrombocytopenia increases the risk of excessive and uncontrolled bleeding.

As inflammation is a feature the body uses to respond to crises, different parts of the body can be inflamed resulting in different symptoms. When the muscles become inflamed(myoscitis), the patient feels weak and the pain in the muscles would increase the content of muscle enzymes within the blood. When vasculitis occurs as a result of inflamed blood vessels, the site (skin, internal organ or the nerve the blood vessel supplies blood to) would have an isolated injury blocking the movement and circulation of blood through these inflamed vessels. When blood is shunted from these regions, there would be depletion of oxygen in that area causing ischemia.

It is often rare for the heart muscles to be affected and become inflamed so as to cause carditis. Young women with SLE when the blood vessels supplying blood to the heart (coronary artery) is deeply affected, there is an significant increase in the risk of heart attacks.

Pleuritis can cause aggravation in breathing as a result of the pain accompanying the inflammation. With time, the entire respiratory region would be engulfed causing other symptoms like coughing chest pain, laboured breathing, and changes in certain body positions.

When the kidney becomes inflamed in Systemic Lupus Erythematosus, a form of lupus called lupus nephritis occurs. This is a condition wherein proteins are found in urine along with the occurrence of hypertension, fluid retention, and subsequently, kidney failure. Without proper treatment, fatigue and pedal oedema can occur. When the kidney fails, dialysis would have to be introduced immediately to ensure proper cleansing of the blood from accumulated waste and toxic products.

Neural and many other nervous changes can occur in the brain leading to certain changes in the patient's personality, psychosis, coma or seizures. Neurologic form of lupus causes damages in the different units that make up the body's nervous system and can be identified as weakness, tingling and numbness of the associated parts of the nervous system connected to the affected area. Lupus cerebritis is a condition of the patient when the brain is fully affected.

Raynaud's phenomenon is seen in patients with SLE wherein the blood vessels of the upper and lower extremities experience spasmic waves when exposed to cold and this in turn compromises the supply of blood to the extremities. This blood shunt would cause the skin around the exposed area to become numb with pain, whitish, and maybe bluish coloration

LUPUS DIET

What is an anti-inflammatory diet?

Diets will always come and go but a disease state such as inflammation caused by Lupus will last forever if not tackled immediately. One can shift his or her lifestyle or diet plan from less inflammatory to anti-inflammatory. There are many tools that can be used to combat the lupus disease but the most powerful which does not come from a pharmacy is obtained right from your neighborhood grocery store.

Given that inflammation is the first sign of the onset of this disease, there is a need to reduce inflammation so as to enable the you live as near a normal life as possible. As such, diets targeted at reducing inflammation are key to well being when you have Lupus. In addition, use of anti-inflammatory diets will help you avoid any potential health issues that would arise from prolonged exposure to chronic inflammation.

When the symptoms of inflammation are reduced or eliminated entirely through adopting an anti-inflammatory diet, there could also be an opportunity to reduce the intake of prescription medication and this will allow you to avoid the additional side effects which can come from prolonged use of drugs.

Within the body, inflammation is the method through which the body fights illness, protects sensitive areas from further injury and harm and heals wounds. However when this natural and healthy response goes wrong the symptoms are painful and often debilitating.

When you follow anti inflammatory diet plan, your goals are to cut down on meals that start off inflammation and increase consumption of diets capable of healing damage already within the body. The ultimate end in using this type of diet is the emphasis which is laid on the need to consume whole unprocessed foods, omega-3 supplements, mono- or unsaturated fats such as avocado and olive oil, vegetables with no starch, limiting the consumption of refined sugar and grains.

If you follow an anti-inflammatory diet, symptoms associated with the inflammation are controlled or reduced to a bare minimum. The need for medication is not to be neglected but research has shown that a combination of the right diet and medications not only helps in reducing inflammation but also countering the effects that comes with the medications. This diet plan is not a guaranteed magic cure but rest assured that the flares you encounter/experience would reduce and the pain would go down by a few notches.

As a widely regarded diet plan, you will have relief from inflammation alongside the reduction of the simultaneous occurrence of other inflammatory diseases. The diet requires you replace refined sugar filled foods with vegetables, fruits and nutrient-rich whole foods. You will increase the amount of anti-oxidants you consume as these molecules are reactive within food, clearing out free radicals/oxidants.

Free radicals are those molecules that appear within the body when certain foods are consumed and digested by the body and they are capable of damaging cells and further increasing the body's risk and tendencies towards certain diseases. Many new diet plans are applying the basic principles of this diet plan; for example the Mediterranean diet requires you to use grain, fish, and monounsaturated fats which are all good for the heart. Using these ingredients and foods, can reduce inflammation in the cardiovascular system which curtails the effects of the disease in the system.

Before one can adopt this diet as part of your new lifestyle, there are several decisions and life changing goals you nee to accepted.

They include:

-consumption of varieties of fruits and vegetables
-complete elimination of junk/fast food in one's diet schedule
-elimination of sugary and soda beverages
-creating well planned shopping lists that will make handy health filled meals and snacks
-carrying snacks that are anti-inflammatory in content
-increasing the quantity of water consumed daily
-starting and remaining within the daily recommended calorific level

-use of supplements that are anti-inflammatory such as turmeric and omega-3
-regular exercise
-increasing your sleep cycle so as to help your body in its healing process

What food groups should you include?

Food groups that need be included in your diet need to have vitamins and enzymes and be raw. Prepare diets that are well balanced containing anti oxidants. Examples of such include green leafy vegetables, fruits. Antioxidants help to restore the body's cellular heath and as well flavonoids that are anti-inflammatory.

With this said, you should clean out your pantry and refrigerator and remove the tempting foods which are on the "to avoid list." Replace them with healthy alternatives. You can try some delicious ant-inflammatory smoothies/juices if you tend to find it difficult in consuming certain portions of leafy green vegetables.

When planning what to put on your plate, a good rule of thumb is to aim to make half to two thirds of it vegetables that are non starchy such as summer squash, cauliflower, greens of all kinds, beets even mushrooms. These vegetables will balance your gut fiber and are going to act as powerful antioxidants in your system with continuous consumption.

Chard is a good green vegetable as they contain high quantities of vitamin A and C which are good anti oxidants, and also have Vitamin K that helps to protect your brain from any oxidative stress due to the presence of free radicals roaming around your system. This can also serve to protect you from the occurrence of Vitamin K deficiency which is commonly associated with Lupus disease.

Another great food to add into your diet regularly is Bok Choy (Chinese Cabbage). This cabbage is an excellent of minerals, vitamins and also an antioxidant. Researchers have detected about 70 substances made of phenolic antioxidants and one of which is hydroxycinnamic acids that particularly scavenges for free radicals. This commonly found vegetable can be used to prepare different dishes which are not Chinese dishes so you can be versatile and not be restricted when you are preparing dishes with this vegetable.

You can also eat cold water fish especially the kinds that are fatty such as tuna, salmon, anchovies, herring, sardines and mackerel. You can also substitute eating these fishes with taking at least 1500mg daily of omega-3 supplement if you do not like fish.

For grains, focus on intact whole grains such as bulgur wheat, brown rice, quinoa etc rather than having to load up on bread, whole crackers, or tortillas. Use nix flour and limit or even reduce the use of other flour based foods.

Foods you can eat but with moderation includes meats, poultry and oily fish.

Other foods that would serve as good choices for an anti inflammatory diet include:

-Dark grapes
-Vegetables which are nutrient-dense like cauliflower and broccoli
-Green tea
-lentils and beans
-fruits such as oranges, cherries, blue and black berries, strawberries
-dark and leafy greens such as kale, spinach and collards
-Tomatoes
-olives, avocado and coconut
-extra virgin olive oil
-dark chocolate
-pine nuts, pistachios
-almonds, cinnamon, turmeric
- Walnuts, spices and herbs

What food groups should you avoid?

Many research studies have shown that certain ingredients in beverages and food can instigate inflammatory effects. Consumption of unhealthy foods will contribute to weight gain which is a high risk factor with regards to starting off inflammation as well.

Fatty acids are major problem, these same fats make up almost about 95% content of our diet and the body sees them as an intruder and it sets off inflammation in response. High cholesterol levels in the system can contribute to inflammation. Thus, when on this diet, avoid saturated fats because they cause an increase in your body's cholesterol levels. Foods that contain this type of fats include garlic, vegetable oils like corn oil, sunflower oil which has a high content of omega-6, red meat, canned foods, processed meat, butter, creamed soups and sauces, baked dairy products that are high in fat, alfalfa sprouts, and animal fat. Alfalfa sprouts has been reported to cause a lupus associated syndrome and lupus flares.

Avoid the intake of soda, beverages sweetened with sugar or natural sweeteners and sugary drinks. When you are on a diet with high sugar content, you will experience an elevation in your blood level of an inflammatory marker, haptogobin. This elevated level indicates your body's gradual shift into a chronic inflammatory state. Not only that, a continuous increase would indicate the presence of already manifested diseases like diabetes, stroke, obesity and heart attack.

Other foods to avoid include:

-processed meat such as sausage, hot dogs and snack foods such as crackers and chips
- White pasta, white potatoes, desserts like candy, cookies and ice cream
-vegetable oil, soybean oil and gluten from store bought bread
 -Ingestion of alcohol
-consumption of too much of refined carbohydrates such as pastries, white bread etc
-Consumption of French fries and other trans fats found in fried foods
-Red meat as found in burgers and steaks
-shortening, margarine and lard

Some of these foods may be challenging when it comes to implementing them into your diet plan. At first, you will see it as a difficult task to achieve but just like other diet plans, with persistence and perseverance, you can include the right food groups and exclude the ones to avoid. Over time, you will notice a steady decrease in the inflammatory symptoms and chronic pain you experience and an ultimate improvement in your overall health.

RECIPES

Breakfast

Cherry coconut porridge

INGREDIENTS

Coconut shavings

9 teaspoons of raw cacao

Pinch of stevia

Frozen or fresh cherries

3-4cups of drinking coconut milk

12 teaspoons of chia seed

Maple syrup

Dark chocolate shavings

11//2 cups of oats

DIRECTIONS

Using a saucepan, combine together the whole oats, stevia, raw cacao and the drinking coconut milk. Mix well before you place it on a medium heat and bring to boil. Allow to simmer over the medium heat until the oats become completely cooked. When properly cooked, pour it into a bowl and top it off with some maple syrup, dark chocolate and coconut shavings, and cherries to taste.

Amaranth Porridge with Pecan Toppings

INGREDIENTS

1/4 teaspoon of ground cloves

1 cup of water

½ spoon of nutmeg

1 spoon of cinnamon

2 large pears

1 cup of amaranth (uncooked)

1/2 tablespoon of maple syrup

1 cup of 2% unsweetened milk

1 teaspoon of ginger (ground)

½ teaspoon of salt to taste

For topping

2 teaspoon of maple syrup

3 tablespoons of pieces of pecan

1½ cup of Greek yoghurt

DIRECTIONS

Preheat your oven (4000C). While the oven is preheating, wash, rinse and drain the amaranth. Mix this amaranth with salt, milk and water and bring it to boil. Reduce it to simmer by reducing the heat to low. Allow to simmer at this level of heat for 28 minutes or until you notice the amaranth has become well cooked and becomes soft.

Ensure there is still some liquid left when the amaranth is soft. Remove it and let it sit for 7 to 12 minutes so that the amaranth can thicken. If you wish, you can thin its texture by adding a little bit of more milk. In another plate, toss the toppings together, that is to say, the maple syrup and spices. Roast this mixture in a pan for up to 20 minutes or till the pears become tender and soft. Stir this mixture into about ¾ of cooling porridge. Spread about half of the Greek yoghourt on the porridge containing the roasted pecans and then place atop it the remaining pieces of pears.

Sweetened Protein Potato

INGREDIENTS

1 sliced small banana

1/2 cup of blueberries

3 pre-baked small sweet potato

1/2 cup of raspberries

2 servings of protein powder

Optional Toppings:

Hemp hearts

Cacao nibs

Your favourite seeds / nut butter

Chia seeds

DIRECTIONS

If your prebaked sweet potato has not been fleshed, do so after which you mash using a fork inside a medium plate. Add the protein powder and stir in gradually until everything is properly combined. Place the blueberries, banana slices and raspberries in a layer format one after each other has been exhausted. Use any additional favourite toppings and simply dig in.

Blueberries and Almonds in Overnight Oats

INGREDIENTS

11/4 cup of whole coconut milk

12 teaspoons of sliced almonds

2 tablespoons of maple syrup

⅓ cup of yogurt

¾ cup old-fashioned oats

½ cup of blueberries

1 pint mason jar

DIRECTIONS

Mix the syrup and milk using a small bowl. Use less quantity of the milk if you want your oatmeal to be thicker. Pour this mixture into a mason jar containing the oats. Cover the jar tightly and allow to stay in the refrigerator overnight. In the morning, remove it from the refrigerator and top the meal with blueberries, your yoghourt and some of the almonds.

Hash Turkey Apple Breakfast.

INGREDIENTS

To prepare the meat

1 teaspoon of cinnamon

3 teaspoon of coconut oil

1 pound of turkey

Salt

To prepare the hash

1 teaspoon cinnamon

1 onion

¾ teaspoon powdered ginger

1 large zucchini

½ teaspoon turmeric

2 cups spinach or greens of choice

2 cups of diced butternut squash

1 large apple, peeled, cored, and chopped

½ teaspoon dried thyme

1 tablespoon coconut oil

½ cup shredded carrots

½ teaspoon garlic

Salt

DIRECTIONS

Over a medium heat, warm 3 teaspoon of coconut oil using a skillet. Remove about 2 teaspoon of the melted coconut oil. In the skillet, cook the ground turkey until it becomes brown. While cooking, season it with the thyme, a pinch of salt and some cinnamon. Transfer to a clean plate. Place the removed 2 teaspoons of coconut oil into the same skillet. Add onions and sauté the oil for 21/2 minutes until the onions becomes soft. Add the carrots, apple, frozen squash and some zucchini. Cook this until the veggies just become soft. When soft, add the spinach and continue stirring until it becomes wilted. Add the removed cooked turkey, stir and taste for salt. Let it cool before you refrigerate it in a sealed container or you can enjoy it fresh from the skillet.

Green Shakshuka

INGREDIENTS

Salt

2 tablespoons harissa

¾ teaspoon coriander

Chopped fresh parsley, as needed for serving

Freshly ground black pepper

2 minced garlic cloves

1 seeded and minced jalapeño

Red-pepper flakes

2 tablespoons extra-virgin olive oil

1 pound spinach

1 teaspoon dried cumin

½ cup vegetable broth

8 large eggs

1 minced onion

Chopped fresh cilantro, as needed for serving

DIRECTIONS

Preheat your oven up to 350F. On a medium heat, heat the extra virgin olive oil in a medium sized skillet. Sauté your onions inside the oil for 4 minutes. After which you add jalapeño, sauté it then add the garlic and sauté again for another one minute. Add the spinach, add salt pepper, coriander and harissa to season it and cook till it becomes properly wilted. Next, transfer this into the food processor bowl and blend this until it becomes coarse. Puree the broth alongside until it becomes thick and smooth. Clean the skillet with a paper towel and grease using a cooking spray that is non-stick. Transfer the blended spinach into the pan and make 6-8 wells using a wooden spoon. Into each of the wells, crack in the eggs. Place the skillet into the oven and bake it till the egg white become set fully with the yolks a little jiggly. After about 22 minutes, remove from the oven and sprinkle some of the cilantro, parsley, shakshuka and the red-pepper flakes. Serve immediately.

Lupus Anti-Inflammatory Porridge

INGREDIENTS

1/4 cup of unsweetened toasted coconut

2 tablespoon of hemp seeds

1/2 teaspoon of cinnamon

A pinch of ground black pepper

2 tablespoon of whole chia seeds)

1/4 cup of coconut milk

1/4 cup of roasted almond butter

3/4 cup of unsweetened almond milk

1 tablespoon of extra virgin coconut oil

1/4 cup of walnut or pecan halves

1/2 - 1 teaspoon of freshly grated turmeric

DIRECTIONS

Chop the walnuts roughly and roast in a hot pan along with the hemp seeds and flaked coconut. Ensure you toss a few times so the nuts don't get burnt and roast until they become fragrant. Set aside in a bowl. Mix and heat the almond and coconut milk together inside a saucepan. Bring to boil before you take it off the heat. Set aside. Mix in the almond butter, chia seeds, the back pepper and coconut oil until they become well combined. Set this aside for about 8 minutes after which you add half of the roasted nuts. Mix the cinnamon with the turmeric powder and spoon it over the porridge. Top off with the roasted mix that is remaining. You can eat it immediately or store it in your fridge for up to 2 days using a tight container.

Vegetable Scramble Wrap

INGREDIENTS

10 inch wheat flour tortilla

6 teaspoons of red onions, chopped

6 teaspoons of green pepper, chopped

1 cup of liquid egg

DIRECTIONS

Using a cooking spray that is non-stick, grease your skillet and place it over a medium heat. Soften your onion and pepper after which you add the liquid egg. Continue to cook while ensuring you stir continuously. When it gets cooked to your liking, spoon it into wheat flour tortilla, roll it up and enjoy. You can also take some grapefruit juice or about 4 ounces of hot brewed tea along with it.

Egg Muffins

INGREDIENTS

Freshly ground black pepper

6 eggs

Salt to taste

Water

For serving

1 large ripe avocado

½ teaspoon of runny honey

1 tablespoon of lemon juice

1 finely chopped scallion

1 cup of chopped flat leaf parsley

DIRECTIONS

Preheat your oven to 375F and grease your muffin pan lightly with extra virgin olive oil. Ensure each hole is coated properly. Place this in the oven and whisk your eggs. Add in some pepper and salt to taste with about 2 teaspoon of water.

Pour the egg mixture into the heated muffin pan up to halfway, and top off with your desired ingredients. Bake this until it becomes golden and is thoroughly cooked. While it is baking, prepare your salsa by dicing your avocado properly after which you mix it with the parsley and scallion inside a large bowl. Balance the acidity with a little honey and some lemon juice. Add salt to taste. When the muffins are golden and are properly baked, leave it to cool for 2 minutes after which you serve with the salsa.

The Five Ingredient Pumpkin Thai Soup

INGREDIENTS

Two 15 ounce cans pumpkin puree

1 large sliced red chili pepper,

32 ounces of vegetable broth,

6 teaspoons of red curry paste

13.5 ounce can of coconut milk,

Cilantro to garnish

DIRECTIONS

Cook the paste of red curry over a medium heat using a saucepan large enough to contain the mixture. Continue to cook it until it becomes fragrant where after, you add the puree and the vegetable broth. Continue to stir until it is cooked for about 4 minutes. As soon as it bubbles, add all the coconut milk ensuring to reserve 3 teaspoons. Continue to cook for 5 minutes after which you then scoop it into bowls. Use the cilantro to garnish if desired after you drizzle the set aside 3 teaspoons and chilli pepper over the soup.

Tuna Salad

INGREDIENTS

Salt and pepper to taste

6 tsp of minced red onion

1/4 cup chopped kalamata or mixed olives

2 large vine-ripened tomatoes

3 tsp of chopped fire roasted red bell peppers

1/4 cup of mayonnaise

2 tbsp of chopped fresh basil

1 tbsp of fresh lemon juice

1 tbsp of capers

2.5 oz cans of drained tuna

DIRECTIONS

Combine all the ingredients except the tomatoes in a large bowl. Stir until they become properly combined after which you slice in the tomatoes in shapes of six's making sure you do not cut through rather you pry it open gently. Now scoop the salad mixture into the centre of each tomato and serve.

Kale Caesar Salad and Grilled Chicken Wrap

INGREDIENTS

½ one minute cooked coddled egg

1/8 cup of fresh lemon juice

2 large tortillas

6 cups bite sized curly kale

1/2 teaspoon Dijon mustard

1 cup quartered cherry tomatoes,

Salt and freshly ground black pepper to taste

 1 clove of minced garlic

3/4 cup finely shredded Parmesan cheese

8 ounces thinly sliced grilled chicken,

1/8 cup of extra virgin olive oil

1 teaspoon agave

DIRECTIONS

Mix half of the egg, agave, garlic, extra virgin olive oil, garlic and mustard in a bowl. Whisk the content f the bowl so a s to form dressing. Add salt and pepper to taste. Next, mix in the quartered tomatoes, thinly sliced chicken and the kale. Toss it properly so as to coat the previously formed dressing. Add a little of the parmesan. On a flat table, place your flatbreads, spread the salad evenly on the wraps before sprinkling each wrap with the parmesan. Roll it up, slice into two then eat it up immediately.

Roasted Red Pepper And Sweet Potato Soup

INGREDIENTS

1 tsp of salt

1 tsp ground coriander

2 chopped medium onions,

4 oz diced green chiles

2 tsp of ground cumin

12 oz roasted red peppers with reserved juice

3 – 4 cups peeled and cubed sweet potatoes

4 oz cubed cream cheese

2 tbsp of minced fresh cilantro

1 tbsp of lemon juice

4 cups vegetable broth

2 tbsp olive oil

DIRECTIONS

Heat the olive oil over medium heat and cook the onions in it until it becomes soft. Add and cook for 2 minutes, the coriander, cumin, salt to taste, green chiles and the red peppers. Pour in the reserved red pepper juice along with the broth and cubed potatoes.

Allow it to boil before you bring the heat down to low, then cover the soup pot. Continue to cook on low heat for 13 minutes after which you add the lemon juice and minced cilantro. Continue to stir then set it aside after 1 minute to cool. Blend half of this soup with the cheese, making sure you puree until the mixture becomes very smooth. Pour t back to the other half in the pot. Heat the mixture again and season with salt if need be.

Smoked Salmon Potato Tartine

INGREDIENTS

Potato Tartine:

2 tbsp of clarified butter

1 large grated russet potato

Pepper and salt to taste

Toppings:

1/2 finely minced garlic clove,

Zest of half a lemon

2 tbsp drained capers

Smoked salmon, thinly sliced

1 1/2 tbsp of finely minced chives

2 tbsp finely chopped red onion

1/2 finely chopped hardboiled egg,

4 ounces of softened goat cheese

DIRECTIONS

In a small bowl assemble and combine thoroughly, the s=zest, goat cheese and garlic. Add pepper and salt to taste before you add the chives. Stir for 30 seconds before you set it aside. Use salt to season the egg and the red onions finely chopped. Set aside. Squeeze the grated potato to remove excess liquid before you season it with pepper and salt then toss. Heat the butter over medium heat and add the grated potato.

Form a rough large circle with the help of a spatula and press the mixture using the back of your spoon to compress it. Cover this and cook on a low heat until it becomes yellowish or golden brown. Flip to the other side and do the same thing until it becomes crispy and golden brown. Allow to cool on a rack. When cool, spread the goat cheese on the top, follow it with smoked salmon and then the mixture of egg, red onions and capers. Cut out the tartine in wedges and serve immediately.

Red Lentil and Squash Curry Stew

INGREDIENTS

4 cups of broth

1 chopped sweet onion,

1/2 tsp of salt & black pepper

1 cup of red lentils

1 tbsp curry powder

1 tsp extra virgin olive oil

3 cups of cooked butternut squash

3 minced garlic cloves

1 cup of greens of preferred choice

DIRECTIONS

Use a large pot to sauté the onions and garlic inside the olive oil. Add the curry powder and stir after heating the onions on low heat for about 4 minutes. Add the lentils and the broth of your choice into the pot and stir till it boils. Continue to cook on low heat for another 9 minutes after which you add you squash and your preferred greens. Cook on medium heat for 7 minutes. Season with pepper and salt, then serve.

Buddha Bowl with Orange, Avocado, Kale and Wild Rice

INGREDIENTS

For the Rice

Freshly ground black pepper and Salt to taste

3 cups water

2 tbsp rice vinegar

1 cup of wild rice

1 minced garlic clove,

1 tbsp chopped fresh mint

2 tbsp extra-virgin olive oil

Toppings

Freshly ground black pepper and Salt to taste

2 hard-boiled eggs

1 bunch of roughly chopped kale,

6 tsp of olive oil

¼ cup of pomegranate seeds

¼ cup pumpkin seeds

1 segmented orange

1 tbsp of rice vinegar

½ sliced avocado,

DIRECTIONS

Make the rice by stirring it with broth and garlic. Allow it to simmer on medium heat until it boils. When it just boils, reduce the heat to low and continue to cook it till its tender. Allow the rice to cook before you toss in olive oil, salt, vinegar, pepper and mint. Set this aside.

Make the toppings by tossing the kale in a bowl along with olive oil and vinegar. Divide the cooked rice into two equal parts and top each with the kale toppings. Place on each half, about 6 teaspoons of pomegranate, half of the sliced avocado and segmented oranges, the boiled egg and 6 teaspoons of pumpkin seeds. Season again with pepper and salt after which you serve.

Glowing Spiced Lentil Soup

INGREDIENTS

1 1/2 tsp ground cumin

1 1/2 tablespoons extra-virgin olive oil

140 grams of rinsed and drained uncooked red lentils,

280 grams of large diced onion

1 package baby spinach

Cayenne pepper, to taste

2 large minced garlic cloves,

1 can of full-fat coconut milk

2 teaspoons ground turmeric

1/2 tsp cinnamon

15-ounce can diced tomatoes

875 mL of vegetable broth

Freshly ground black pepper and Salt to taste

1/4 tsp ground cardamom

2 tsp fresh lime juice

DIRECTIONS

Mix the oil, garlic and onion in a large pot. Sauté on medium heat until the onions soften, add the turmeric, cardamom and the cinnamon until everything becomes properly combined. Cook it until it becomes fragrant.

Add the coconut milk, broth, salt and pepper to taste, plenty of cayenne pepper, lentils and the tomatoes. Stir and increase the heat to high until it boils. On boiling, reduce to medium and allow it to simmer while open until the lentils are tender. At this moment, turn the heat off and stir in the spinach into the pot till it wilts. Add fresh juice of lime to taste and check for salt and pepper. Serve in bowls with lime wedges.

Golden Sun-Dried Tomato Red Lentil Pasta.

INGREDIENTS

2 large handfuls of baby kale

1/4 cup of olive oil

1/2 cup of oil packed sun-dried tomatoes

8 ounce box red lentil pasta

1 chopped sweet onion,

1 tbsp of dried oregano

2 tsp of ground turmeric

1 can of fire roasted tomatoes

6 minced cloves garlic

1 tbsp apple cider vinegar

1 tbsp of dried basil

Salt and pepper

For topping

Toasted pine nuts

Nutritional yeast,

Grated parmesan

DIRECTIONS

Heat and simmer the olive oil using a medium pot on a medium heat. As soon as the oil starts simmering, sauté the onions till it becomes soft. Add the basil, minced garlic, turmeric, oregano, pepper and salt to taste.

Stir and cook it until it becomes fragrant. Crush the tomatoes and add it and the juice into the pot. Mix in the vinegar and the sun-dried tomatoes. Simmer for 14 minutes after which you can puree the sauce if you wish in a blender. Add the baby kale and cook for 3 minutes. While boiling, prepare your pasta in salted water according to the manufacturer's direction, Serve with herbs or cheese.

Anti-inflammatory Chicken Wrap

INGREDIENTS

For the chicken:

Few shakes of dried oregano

Few shakes of lemon pepper

3 teaspoons of olive oil

Few shakes of garlic powder

2 bone-in chicken breasts

Baking sheet

For the Greek salad

6 teaspoons of hummus for each wrap

1 cup of sliced cherry tomatoes,

Olive oil

½ cup of sliced and halved cucumber slices

6 teaspoons of kalamata olives

4 cups of chopped romaine

A cup of feta cheese

¼ cup of red onion

Whole wheat wraps

Red wine vinegar

DIRECTIONS

To cook the chicken, first preheat your oven to 375F. Use a foil to line your sheet with foil and oil it lightly with a drizzle of 1½ teaspoon of the olive oil. Carefully place the chicken breasts atop the now oiled foil.

Add pepper and salt to season it before adding a few shakes of the lemon pepper, dried oregano to season the breasts. Oil the breasts again with about 1½ teaspoon of the olive oil, place in the preheated oven and bake for 39 minutes to make sure the chicken becomes thoroughly cooked. You can choose to either use it up immediately or store some leftovers for the wraps. This baked quantity should just be enough to prepare about 4 wraps that will be large in size.

Prepare the salad by placing the romaine first into a small bowl after which you top it off with the feta cheese, sliced cucumbers, red onions that is well diced, some olives and the cherry tomatoes. Add on top of these a few shakes of the oregano and dress this using vinegar in such a way as to go twice around the bowl. Continue dressing with olive oil but this time going one turn round the bowl. Stir this and add more seasonings if need be.

Make the wrap by spreading the 6 teaspoons of hummus unto your desired wrap. Place the chicken slices on the wraps to top it followed with heaping a large portion of the salad

Roll the wraps and eat up.

Butternut Squash and Roasted Carrot Soup

INGREDIENTS

5-6 cups vegetable stock

1 1/2 lb of carrots,

1/2 cup shallot

1/2 tsp pepper

1 1/2 pounds butternut squash,

3 tsp of grated turmeric

1 tsp of Kosher's salt

1 tsp of grated ginger

3 tbsp olive oil divided into portions

GARNISHING:

Coconut milk

Roasted chickpeas

Cilantro

DIRECTIONS

Turn on your oven and preheat it to 400F. Dice your shallot, cut the carrots into 1/2 inch piece, then peel and dice your squash. Place the carrots and squash into your baking pan and drop 2 tbsp of the olive oil on the veggies in a drizzle form. Add salt to taste.

Then, place in the oven and roast this until it becomes tender on ricked with fork and this should take 25-30 minutes. While the veggies are roasting, heat the other tablespoon of olive oil in a soup pot large enough to contain the meal. Use the oil to sauté the grated turmeric, diced shallot and the grated ginger till it becomes fragrant to perceive which should take about 1 minute. Continue to stir when you sauté so that they will not burn. Add into the stock. Place on medium heat, don't cover the pot and bring it to boil. When it just begins to boil, cover the pot, reduce the heat to low and allow it to simmer while the veggies are still in the oven. When the veggies are well roasted, add it into the pot, mix to combine properly. Ladle this mixture into a food processor then puree it on high speed. Pour this into the pot when done and heat again till it's ready to be served. Add in seasoning if need be. Garnish with some coconut milk, cilantro and the chickpeas. Enjoy!

Dinner

Quinoa & Turkey Stuffed with Bell Peppers

INGREDIENTS

1.25 pounds of ground extra lean turkey

3 large yellow peppers

1 cup of chopped fresh spinach

1 cup of diced mushrooms

1 cup of tomato sauce

1/4 cup sweet onion, diced

1 cup of dry quinoa

½ tablespoon of garlic, minced

1 cup of chicken broth

9x13 baking pan

Cooking spray

DIRECTIONS

Preheat the oven to 400. In a small saucepan, start the quinoa and cook according to the manufactures direction which should be for 15 minutes. Meanwhile, place a little butter or olive oil in a pan and use it to sauté your vegetables for 5 minutes.

Place the garlic and turkey in the pan containing the sautéed vegetables. Allow this to cook on a high-medium heat till the turkey has become thoroughly cooked. Next, pour in ½ of the broth along with the tomato sauce. Allow these to simmer over the medium heat till you cook off excess water in the pan. The turkey should be properly cooked at this point. Preheat your oven to about 400F. Wash and prepare your peppers by cutting them in half portions. Clean the insides of the peppers by removing the seeds and the stem. Lightly oil your pan using the spray. Place the cleaned peppers inside it facing the cut open side up. When the quinoa is cooked, pour it into the pan containing the vegetables and the turkey. Stir this mixture to properly mix them and then pour these into the peppers making sure to properly stuff the peppers nicely to the brim using the mixture. If you will want to use cheese, cover the mixture with it at this point in such a way that it is barely covered. If you use too much of the cheese, it can make your oven become super messed up. The remaining broth should be poured into the base of the baking pan in such a way that it doesn't cover the peppers but rather around them. Place a foil over the pan to cover it properly. This makes sure the heat stays within the pan to bake the peppers and turkey mixture properly. Bake inside the preheated oven at 400F for 35-40 minutes before you remove from the oven. Eat it up while warm as they taste so good that warm.

Curried Potatoes And Poached Eggs

INGREDIENTS

1 inch fresh ginger

4 large eggs

2 russet potatoes

2 tablespoon of curry powder

2 cloves garlic

1 tablespoon of olive oil

15 oz can tomato sauce

OPTIONAL

1/2 bunch fresh cilantro

DIRECTIONS

Wash your potatoes properly after which you then cut into them 3/4-inch cubes. Place these cubed potatoes inside a large pot, cover with water and heat on high-medium heat. Bring it to boil for about 5-6 minutes so as to make them tender when pierced with a fork.

While the potatoes are boiling, prepare the sauce. Use a vegetable peeler to peel the ginger or you can scrape the skin off with the help of the side of a spoon. Grate about one inch of ginger using a small holed cheese grater after which you mince the garlic.

Into a large, deep skillet, add in the ginger, garlic, and olive oil. Sauté the ginger and garlic over medium low heat for about 1-2 minutes or until they become soft and fragrant. Add in the curry powder to the skillet and sauté for about a minute more so as to toast the spices.

Add the tomato sauce to the skillet and mix properly to combine. Increase the heat up to medium and heat the sauce thoroughly. Add salt to taste. Drain the cooked potatoes using a colander and it to the skillet. Continue to stir to ensure they get well coated in the sauce. Add in a couple of tablespoons of water should the mixture seem to be dry or pasty in consistency. Inside the potato mixture, create four small wells or dips and crack in an egg into each of the wells. Cover the skillet with a lid on and let the mixture come up to a simmer. Let the eggs simmer in the sauce for about 6-10 minutes so that they become cooked thoroughly or you can cook if for a less time if you want runny yolks. Serve with chopped fresh cilantro if desired to top it off.

One Pan Lemon Herb Salmon And Zucchini

INGREDIENTS

4 chopped zucchini,

6 teaspoons of olive oil

Freshly ground black pepper and salt to taste

FOR THE SALMON

4 (5-ounce) salmon fillets

1/2 teaspoon dried dill

1/4 teaspoon dried rosemary

2 packed tablespoons of brown sugar,

2 tablespoons chopped fresh parsley leaves

1/4 teaspoon dried thyme

2 tablespoons freshly squeezed lemon juice

1 tablespoon Dijon mustard

2 minced cloves garlic

1/2 teaspoon dried oregano

Freshly ground black pepper and salt to taste

OPTIONAL

Parsley

DIRECTIONS:

Preheat your oven to 400F. Oil your baking sheet lightly using a non stick spray.

Using small sized bowl, whisk together oregano, Dijon mustard, garlic, brown sugar, lemon juice, dill, thyme and rosemary; add pepper and salt to taste after which you set it aside.

On the greased baking sheet, place in a single layer your zucchini after which you drizzle with some olive oil. Thereafter, add pepper and salt to taste. In a single layer, place your salmon. After which you brush each of the salmon fillet with the herb mixture. Cook inside the heated oven until the fish easily flakes when turned with a fork or you can leave it to cook for about 15-17 minutes. Garnish with parsley if desired and serve immediately.

Slow Cooker Turkey Chili

INGREDIENTS

2 (15oz) cans rinsed and drained red kidney beans

1 tablespoon cumin

2 (15 oz) cans tomato sauce

1 pound 99% lean ground turkey

2 (15 oz) cans petite diced tomatoes

2 (15 oz) cans rinsed and drained black beans

2 tablespoons chili powder

1 diced medium onion

1 chopped red pepper

1 (16 oz) drained jar deli-sliced tamed jalapeno peppers

1 chopped yellow pepper

3 teaspoon of olive oil

1 cup frozen corn

Black pepper and salt to taste

Optional toppings

Sour cream/Greek yogurt

Shredded cheese,

Green onions,

Avocado,

DIRECTIONS

Place a skillet over medium heat and heat the olive oil. Heat the turkey in the skillet until it turns brown after which you pour into a slow cooker.

Add the corn, peppers, beans, onion, diced tomatoes, jalapeños, chili powder, tomato sauce and cumin. Add pepper and salt to taste and stir. Use a lid and cover the cooker. Cook on high heat for about 4 hours or if you wish to cook it for a longer time, cook for 6 hours on a low heat for 6 hours. If desired, serve with any of the toppings.

Snacks

Paleo AIP Donut Holes with Tigernuts & Cinnamon

INGREDIENTS

5 teaspoons of honey

1 cup of dried shredded unsweetened coconut flakes

A pinch of Kosher's salt

1/2 teaspoon of pure vanilla powder

4 medjool dates with their pits removed

1/4 cup tigernut flour

1 teaspoon of cinnamon

OPTIONAL COATING:

6 teaspoons of maple or coconut sugar

DIRECTIONS

Use a mini food processor so as to keep making this recipe easy to do as well as involve minimal cleaning. Process your dried coconut using the food processor, for about 25 seconds to 60 seconds so that the oils can be released.

Add the vanilla, sea salt, cinnamon and the ¼ tigernut flour into the processed coconut flakes. Process these again until the mixture becomes properly combined and has a fine texture. Add your dates and continue to process for about 1 minute after which you add your honey. Use your hands and form the mixture into balls after which if you want, you can coat the balls with the sugar. You can enjoy it this way or preferably, freeze it inside an airtight container. If you leave it at room temperature, for a day or two, they will still be okay for eating.

No-Bake Chocolate Chia Energy Bars

INGREDIENTS

70 g chopped dark chocolate

350 g pitted dates

45 g unsweetened shredded coconut

75 g chia seeds

125 g pieces of raw walnut

35 g raw cocoa powder or cocoa powder

50 g oats

Square baking pan

OPTIONAL

1 teaspoon of pure vanilla

1/4 teaspoon of Kosher's salt

DIRECTIONS

Place the pitted dates in your food processor and process. Stop puree and add in the walnuts when you have a thick paste formed. Continue to puree to combine them well.

Next, place the other ingredients into the processor and mix properly till you have dough that is thick. Use parchment paper to line your baking pan, after which you press the mixture unto the pan firmly. At the corners, press it lightly so they don't stick onto the paper when properly baked. Freeze this for about 6-9 hours or you can leave it overnight. Remove the frozen mixture from the pan and cut into 14 pieces. You can continue to freeze it or place it in your fridge stored inside an airtight container.

Berry Freezer Pops

INGREDIENTS

1 cup Strawberries

3 cups Plain low fat yogurt

1 1/2 tbsp Almonds

Small paper cups

DIRECTIONS

Place the almonds and strawberries and in a food processor and puree the mixture to form very small pieces. Add in yogurt and pulse a few times. Equally divide the now formed yogurt mixture in 6 small paper cups. Into each cup, place a popsicle stick in the middle of the yogurt and freeze overnight. Remove from the freezer and peel the paper cup before eating.

Cauliflower Popcorn

INGREDIENTS

4 cups Cauliflower

2 teaspoons of extra virgin olive oil

Salt to Taste

DIRECTIONS

Core and cut the cauliflower into florets and coat with extra virgin olive oil by tossing it. Sprinkle with a generous amount of salt to taste, then roast at 450°F for about 25-30 minutes until they become tender and browned. Drizzle with extra virgin olive oil then serve.

Cottage Cheese Snack

INGREDIENTS

10 quartered Cherry Tomatoes

1/4 cup Low-Fat Cottage Cheese

1/4 teaspoon of dried basil

1/4 teaspoon of pepper

2 1/2 tablespoon of sliced Olives

DIRECTIONS

Cut the cherry tomatoes in half. Stir in the basil and pepper as well as the cottage cheese in a small bowl. Gently stir in the tomatoes and the sliced olives. Serve.

Greek Yogurt Snack

INGREDIENTS

1/4 cup 0% Fat Greek yogurt

1 large sized cucumber

1/4 tsp Cumin

6 sliced Olives

Pepper and Salt

DIRECTIONS

Cut the seeds of the cucumber off and chop into quarters. Stir in the Greek yogurt, cumin, salt and pepper together in a small bowl. Gently stir in olives and cucumber. Then serve.

Superfood High Protein Cacao Bites

INGREDIENTS

1 cup cashews

Sea salt to taste

12 teaspoons of cacao

1 tablespoon vanilla extract

6 teaspoons of ground flaxseeds

4 tablespoons almond milk with vanilla flavouring

1 cup sprouted almonds

OPTIONAL

A scoop of turmeric tonic

1 scoop collagen peptides

1 tablespoon maca powder

DIRECTIONS

Pulse the almond and cashew in your blender until you get n almost flour consistency. Don't allow it to become too fine in texture, so don't pulse the nuts completely to become well ground.

Next, you add the rest of the ingredients except the almond milk. Pulse again to properly mix the ingredients well. At this point add your milk and continue to pulse. Stop the blender when you have a dough formed. Should the dough feel sticky to touch, add 1 tablespoon of the milk then pulse. Add one tablespoon at a time so it doesn't become very sticky to roll into balls. Using about 4 tablespoons, should give the right consistency for the dough. Use your hands to form the dough into small balls after which you coat it with the cocoa powder, coconut flakes and the hemp seeds. Store this using an airtight container inside your freezer if you are not eating it right away. You can store for as long as 7-14 days or even longer while inside your freezer.

Vanilla Energy Bites

INGREDIENTS

3 cups of apple rings, dried

1 cup of apricots, dried

2 vanilla beans,

1 zested lemon with 1 teaspoon reserved

½ juiced lemon

¼ cup of coconut oil

½ cup of coconut, finely shredded

A pinch of Kosher's salt

DIRECTIONS

Get your vanilla beans, sliced it open lengthwise, then scrape the seeds out and reserve it. Add the vanilla bean seeds, lemon juice, apricots, apple rings, lemon zest and coconut oil to a food processor.

Use all the lemon zest less one teaspoon. Puree on high speed to make sure they become thoroughly combined and feels sticky to touch and this should take about 60-120 seconds. Combine the sea salt, shredded coconut and the set aside teaspoon of lemon zest inside a bowl small enough to contain them all. Roll the mixture you processed into small sized balls with your hands, rolling about 6 teaspoons at a time. Coat with the coconut mixture you combined in the small bowl, after which you place it in a plate. After you have formed all into small sized bites, refrigerate these balls for 20-25 minutes before you enjoy it. This hardens the balls. Leave the bites in the fridge till its all finished so that they remained hardened.

* 9 7 8 1 7 2 1 7 0 4 3 7 8 *